The Psoriasis Diet

By

Lynne D M Noble

Independently published

Contents

Dedication

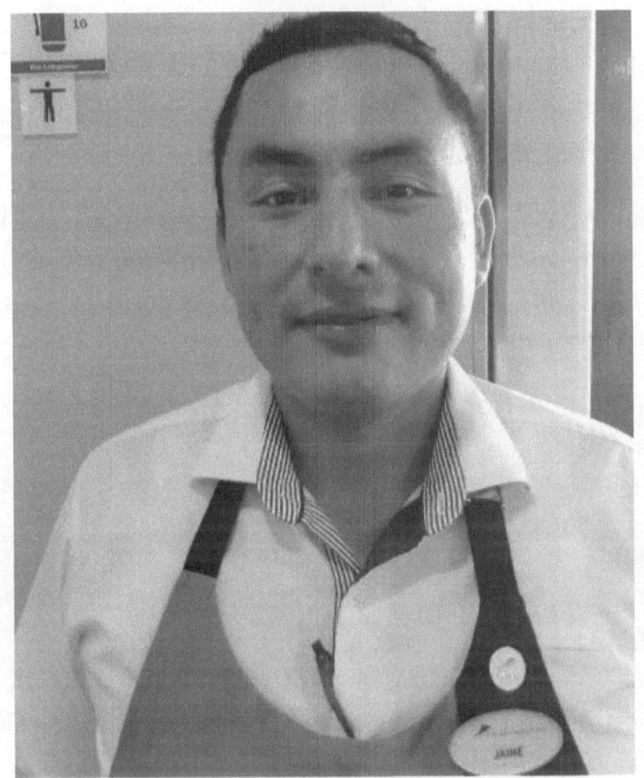

Jaime Luis Cortez Ocsa

from

Callao Peru

Thank you for the interest in my work.

About the Author

Lynne Noble was born in 1953 in Huddersfield, West Yorkshire. From a very early age, Lynne showed an interest in nutrition and genetics avidly reading any books that she could get her hands on at the time.

Initially, Lynne studied orthopaedics but events led her to work with the elderly mentally infirm. Here, her interest in neurodegenerative disorders and pain syndromes developed.

Lynne undertook rigorous programmes of study, completing her Cert Ed., (FE) BSc (Hons) and Adv. Dip Education simultaneously before moving onto her M.Ed.

From there she took further demanding programmes in Human Nutrition, Pharmacology, Neuroscience, Genetics and Immunology. During this time, she was given many prestigious awards for her academic work. It was noted then that Lynne was not afraid of tackling difficult subjects.

She began her law degree but ill health prevented her from pursuing this. However, in this time, she moved from being a foster parent to adoptive parent.

She has been instrumental in setting up projects in the community for disadvantaged groups.

She is a member of the Guild of Health Writers.

Now retired, she lives in a picturesque village in West Yorkshire with her husband. She enjoys gardening, watching her husband bowling and researching.

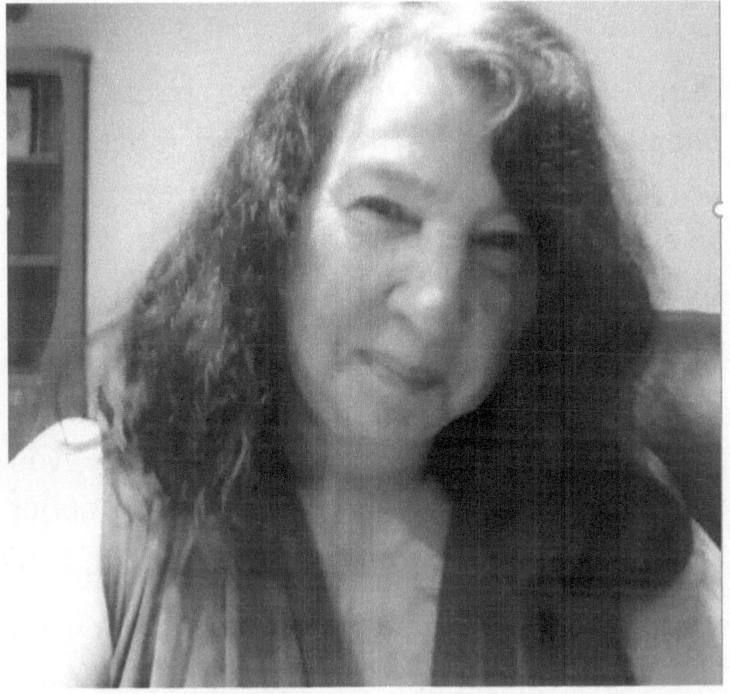

Author Lynne Noble at home

https://quintessentiallylynne.weebly.com/nutritional-medicine.html

Preface

During my lifetime I have come across many people with psoriasis that is so often itchy and disfiguring that many have hidden themselves away in their homes and have socially isolated themselves.

Most people who don't have psoriasis misunderstand the condition believing it to be contagious. Thus, the sufferer is isolated, even further - through lack of understanding - about the condition, from others.

Psoriasis appears to be given low priority when it comes to research and treatment of the condition. There are a number of treatments but the side effects are not acceptable and don't tackle the condition at source. Most individuals who suffer from psoriasis find the application of coal tar products or Anthralin, intolerable. Both are greasy and stain heavily. Not only does the psoriasis sufferers have to deal with disfiguring patches, intolerable itching, flakes of dry skin which get everywhere, but the use of some topical ointments incurs a great deal of extra washing.

The use of topical steroids – while reducing the itch and inflammation – should always be used with caution. Continued use thins the skin. They increase the risk of infection when skin is broken. As psoriasis is a chronic inflammatory disease then topical steroid ointment may be prescribed for long term use.   This is not acceptable either.

On my first trip to the GP accompanying a friend who had psoriasis, she was prescribed Voltarol for the inflammation. On application, it actually increased the inflammatory processes resulting In Intense itching. A return trip to the GP resulted in a prescription for Betnovate – a topical steroid ointment.   My friend was instructed to apply the steroid cream first and once the inflammation had calmed down, to apply the Voltarol. My friend now had an ointment that thinned the skin and an anti-inflammatory that can cause liver damage!

The itching can be so intense that sufferers may scratch plaques until they bleed raising the risk of infection when the skin is broken.

In spite of all this, those individuals who live with psoriasis, in the UK have found that any government assistance that was available to help with the costs generated by this condition, have now been withdrawn.

Psoriasis is a condition which is co-morbid for a number of other conditions. There are a number of underlying processes in common which give us a clue to what is going on.

Many of these processes are amenable to dietary modification as is psoriasis. While there may be a genetic component to psoriasis, by the biggest deciding factor in whether it manifests itself are environmental factors.

It is harder to uncover the environmental factors involved in the manifestation of psoriasis. This condition has a long history which we will look at shortly. Nevertheless, our understanding that psoriasis is the result of chronic inflammation and occurs alongside other specific conditions places us admirably to devise a diet that respond to the underlying processes found in this condition.

This book will take a brief look at the history of psoriasis, including past and current treatments. The processes involved in the development and progression of the condition are also investigated before considering how a bespoke diet can respond to the processes fuelling the disease, thus reducing - or alleviating entirely - the need for medical treatment.

History of Psoriasis

As I have already stated, psoriasis is not a de novo – new disease. If it was then it would be far easier to identify environmental factors that contribute to the manifestation of this condition. However, its history is long. Psoriasis has been found in Egyptian mummies. Clearly, the exposure to constant, penetrating sunlight, that synthesises huge amounts of vitamin D, did not prevent this condition from manifesting itself.

Some of the treatments for psoriasis, in early medicine, included arsenic. This was not found to benefit the sufferer or their condition.

Galen was the first physician who coined the term psoriasis which means 'itch.' His treatments - along with applying arsenic topically - included applying a lotion in which a viper had been boiled. This was not found to be effective, either.

Many treatments were smelly and time-consuming to apply. They were ineffective and caused further irritation. In many respects we have not advanced a great deal in the treatment of psoriasis.

Many treatments involved moisturising the skin and covering in bandages for days. This was supposed to loosen the plaques. However, it did nothing for the underlying processes causing the condition. Nevertheless, one of our more most recent – and unusual therapies - was founded in Turkey. Doctor fish, known as garra rufa, nibble on the psoriatic scales of those who venture into the pools.

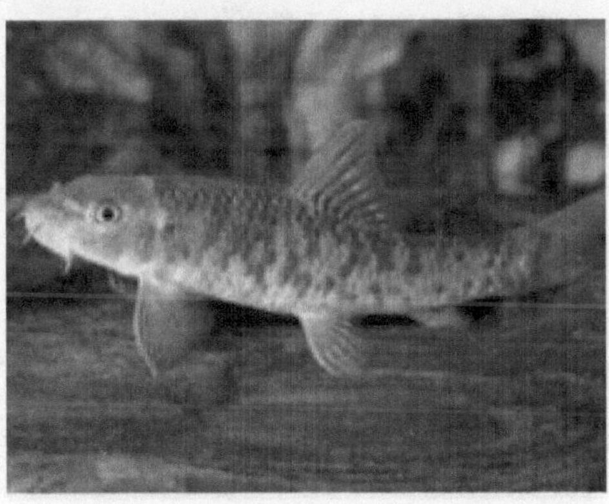

The garra rufa fish nibble on psoriatic plaques smoothing the skin in the process

The association with leprosy – a highly contagious skin condition – was not severed until 1840. Nevertheless, the understanding that psoriasis may be autoimmune in nature did not occur until over one hundred years later when a number of treatments including topical applications, phototherapy and systemic medicine became the main treatments for psoriasis depending on the severity of its manifestation.

We can see that psoriasis has a long history which has resulted in some unusual and mainly ineffective treatments. This leads us neatly into our next chapter which looks at current treatments for this condition

To be an effective treatment we need to not just address the symptoms but the cause underlying the condition. How effective are these treatments in meeting these standards?

Currently prescribed treatments for psoriasis

Treatment for psoriasis falls into three main categories and these are:

- Topical applications
- Light therapy
- Systemic medication

The topical applications include corticosteroids, retinoids and vitamin D analogues.

Vitamin D analogues

The most commonly prescribed vitamin D analogues are Dovonex which comes in a thick ointment for application to the skin and a lotion which can be applied to the scalp. Neither of these products appear to be particularly welcomed by those with psoriasis.

The topical application of Dovonex, while moisturising the skin and helping to loosen the plaques, forms a sticky layer. This attracts anything it comes into contact with. It may be useful for the odd psoriatic plaque that can be covered but it is not practical for whole body use.

In addition, the Dovonex scalp lotion produces quite a greasy look to the hair which has to be washed more frequently than one would probably do without its application.

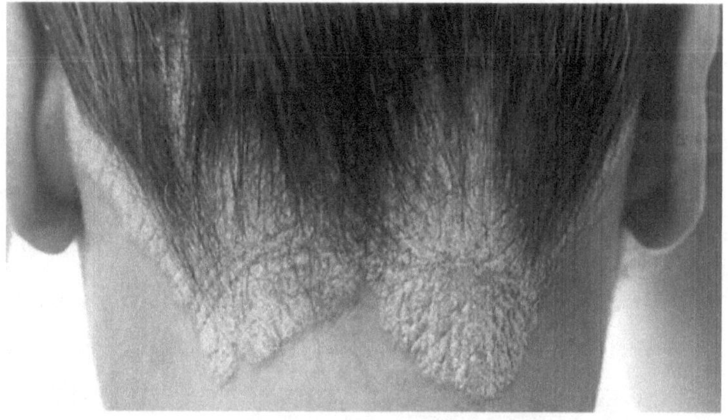

Scalp psoriasis is a distressing condition to say the least.

The idea behind vitamin D analogues is that they will reduce inflammatory responses in the way that vitamin D calms the immune system from over-reacting to stimuli. It helps to slow the overly active skin growth characteristic of psoriasis. Vitamin D has been found to be deficient in many autoimmune disorders. As vitamin D is synthesised from the sun we would expect that those living in sunny climes would be less likely to have psoriasis. Nevertheless, in spite of the fierce and prolonged sunshine in Egypt, the Egyptian mummies were still found to have suffered from psoriasis.

Vitamin D analogues are not generally a popular treatment given the extra washing that appears to go alongside with their use. They do not appear to be effective in tackling psoriasis at root level. Nevertheless, some people may benefit from vitamin D analogues.

Topical corticosteroids

Topical corticosteroids are prescribed frequently for mild to moderate cases of psoriasis. They produce rapid relief from the itching and inflammation that accompanies psoriasis. A few hours after application, the skin can look quite healthy. Nevertheless, this effect does not last unless the steroid cream is used on a regular basis.

The difficulty with any topical corticosteroid such as Betnovate and Eumovate is that they thin the skin over time. As they depress the immune system they are also a risk factor for infection. Systemic steroid use also produces similar reactions but in a more pronounced way. For short term use topical steroids are a useful adjunctive treatment but should not be considered for long term use.

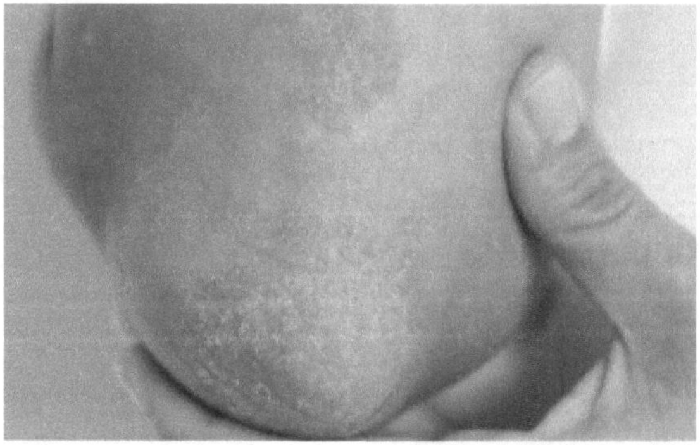

Psoriatic plaques on the elbow which appears to be a very common place for them to appear.

Topical retinoids

Topical retinoids are a vitamin A derivative. They help to decrease inflammation and skin irritation. However, they increase sensitivity to sunlight. Those using topical retinoids are advised to keep out of the sun while they are applying them, otherwise redness and blistering can occur.

Of course, the use of topical retinoids thus deprives individuals, with psoriasis, the benefit of being out in the sun and synthesising vitamin D from the sun's rays.

Salicylic acid

Salicylic acid is an anti- inflammatory that helps reduce the scaling found in psoriasis. Some people find that salicylic acid can initially make the itching worse leading to an itch-scratch-itch cycle. While salicylic acid has some benefits, some people are allergic to it. It can produce rapid swelling of the tissues in susceptible people. As it does not address the root causes of psoriasis, it is normally used as a long term treatment.

Coal tar derivatives

Coal tar derivatives were one of the original treatments proven to work by reducing skin turnover and inflammation. However, coal tar derivatives tend to be smelly and stain clothes. They still do not address the root cause of psoriasis.

Calcineurin Inhibitors

Calcineurin inhibitors reduce the production of a substance known as interleukin-2 that is found in endothelial cells in psoriasis. It also results in the reduced expression of tiny receptors on cells known as   IL-2R. The knock on effect of this is a reduction in T cell activation. T cell infiltration is found in psoriatic lesions.

Anthralin

Anthralin helps to slow skin cell growth but may irritate the skin. In addition, it stains clothing resulting in extra washing.

Moisturisers

Moisturisers are often used to relieve the dry skin that is characteristic of psoriasis. Dry skin is often associated with itching so moisturisers may not only protect the skin from breaking - which is a risk factor for infection – but calm the itching. They may be sticky and build up on clothing. In addition, they don't address the underlying causes of psoriasis. However, they are a useful adjunctive treatment.

Light Therapy as a treatment for Psoriasis

Light therapy which uses broadband UVB is useful for slowing skin turnover, scaling and inflammation. It can be used for problematical single patches involving itching and irritation.

Systemic Medications

Sometimes – where psoriatic plaques are resistant to light therapy or topical applications – systemic medications may be given which are steroid based.

Steroids have a dramatic impact on inflammatory processes but they have a number of unwanted and serious side effects so they are not for long term use. Some of these side effects are:

- An increase in blood sugar levels resulting in a pre-diabetic or diabetic state.
- A marked increase in blood pressure.
- Raised intraocular pressures – therefore not suitable for those with glaucoma

- Muscle wasting
- Extreme emotional fragility
- Insomnia
- Thinning of skin. This would not make them suitable for those with certain connective tissue disorders such as Ehlers Danlos Syndrome.
- Increased risk of infection

This is not a definitive list. Taking steroids should not be taken lightly at any time.

While it is clear that we have come a long way in finding treatments which address the symptoms, many of these may be time consuming, lack effectiveness, result in unwanted side effects and increased personal laundry. Further, they do not address the underlying causes of psoriasis. For those with whole body psoriasis as opposed to a single psoriatic patch, this is unacceptable.

To understand psoriasis, we need to look at the processes involved in the development and progression of this skin condition. In doing so we may find inflammatory pathways, for example, that may be amenable to a bespoke diet.

The next chapter then contains some more in depth material than has currently been found in the first couple of chapters. We touch on the immune system and discover what the difference is between acute and chronic inflammation. This is vital for our understanding of this skin condition. The more we know about the underlying processes, the better equipped we are to address it.

Processes involved in the development and progression of psoriasis

Psoriasis is known to be an autoimmune and chronic inflammatory condition which may be relapsing and remitting in nature.

Psoriasis is often comorbid with a number of connective tissue disorders such as:

- Rheumatoid arthritis
- Systemic lupus erythematosus
- Dermatomyositis
- Scleroderma

Connective tissue diseases are a diverse group of conditions but they are all characterised by the abnormal structure - or functioning - of some of the composition of the connective tissue. The above named connective tissue disorders are also, like psoriasis, autoimmune in origin. Knowing that psoriasis is linked with the above conditions gives us an insight into the underlying processes that come together - and result - in this skin condition known as psoriasis.

One of the processes found in common with these connective tissue disorders and psoriasis is that of angiogenesis. Angiogenesis is not normally talked about when we mention psoriasis but it is an important process in the development of psoriasis. As such it demands a section all to itself. It is to this subject that we shall now turn.

Angiogenesis

Angiogenesis is perhaps better known as the process that occurs during the development of cancerous tumours. Angiogenesis is the formation of new blood vessels from existing ones that will connect to the body's main circulatory system. For this process a substance known as Vascular Endothelial Growth Factor (VEGF) is required. Angiogenesis is generally a pathological process as seen in the development of atherosclerosis, diabetic retinopathy, rheumatoid arthritis, macular degeneration, psoriasis, tumour growth and chronic inflammation.

 As the development and progression of psoriasis also involves the neo-formation of an existing vascular bed, it is prudent to examine what dietary substances can prevent angiogenesis from taking place.

Fortunately, there are many angio-preventative foods and these include:

- fruits
- vegetables
- herbs
- sea foods
- tea
- coffee
- dark chocolate
- Lycopene (lycopene is the antioxidant that gives tomatoes their red colour)
- Genistein – found in soy products
- Epigallocatechin - found in green tea
- Resveratrol – found in red wine
- Kahweol – found in unfiltered coffee
- Oleocanthol and
- Hydroxytyrosol both of which are found in virgin extra olive oil

Beatriz Martinez-Poveda[1], a researcher extolled the virtues of the Mediterranean diet explaining that it contains many angiopreventative foods. As such it is an ideal diet for those with psoriasis to follow. Not only does the diet prevent angiogenesis but it also contains many anti-inflammatory compounds that also contribute to the development and progression of psoriasis. Olive oil – a monounsaturated oil, for example, is a powerful anti-inflammatory and is used liberally in the Mediterranean diet. However, olive oil should be stored well. It should be stored in a cool, dark place to avoid oxidisation. It should never be heated.

Olive oil is very versatile. Use it on salads liberally, add a tablespoon to soups or dip your bread into it as an accompaniment to savoury dishes.

---

[1] Beatriz Martinez-Poveda et al in The Mediterranean Diet, a rich source of angiopreventative compounds in cancer Sept 2019, 11 (8) 2036

Creating a situation where angiogenesis cannot occur is vital. It removes one of the steps that are vital in the development of psoriasis.

Milk has also been found to contain three substances which inhibit angiogenesis. The main inhibitor is lactoferrin. Lactoferrin is a major component of milk fat globules. It contributes to phagocytic removal of damaged cells. It has been found to inhibit tumour formation as well as exhibiting anti-inflammatory activity.

Strangely, lactoferrin is found in tears, human milk – more than bovine milk products- saliva and nasal secretions. As an important multi-functional protein it is found on all mucosal surfaces where it kills staphylococcus aureus. Lactoferrin has been found to be elevated in arthritis, inflammatory bowel disease and periodontitis. It is required to deal with the inflammatory nature of these conditions.

A number of vitamins have essential roles in the prevention of angiogenesis while others aid the process. Clearly, in conditions like psoriasis, we are seeking to prevent angiogenesis from occurring. Vitamins have specific roles in the prevention of angiogenesis. Some suppress VEGF and others may supress the proliferation of endothelium cells.

Endothelial cell adhesion molecules are found in psoriasis. They are antigens which bring about the adhesion of inflammatory cells to endothelium. These cell adhesion molecules may help white blood cells infiltrate psoriatic plaques.

The vitamins that can actually progress angiogenesis are vitamin B1, B12 and B5. While we cannot and should not avoid them since they are required for other processes in the body, it would perhaps be sensible to avoid foods that contain large amounts of these vitamins.

Vitamin B12 is one vitamin that can only be found in animal protein. Vegetarians and vegans have to take supplements in order to avoid vitamin B12 deficiency. Vitamin B12 needs an acidic environment to be separated from its food source in order that it may be utilised in the body. Therefore, those taking antacids for other conditions may be deficient in vitamin B12. It is a vital vitamin for the health of the brain and many other processes in the body. There is a condition known as pernicious anaemia that occurs due to the lack of availability of vitamin B12. Sufferers of pernicious anaemia, In the earlier 1900's, were required to eat up to 2lb of raw liver daily in order to take in the recommended daily allowance of vitamin B12, if they wanted to survive.

Many people supplement vitamin B12 without knowing whether they have a deficiency of this vitamin. It has become one of those fashionable vitamins to take as it appears to enhance both physical and mental energy. Many individuals with symptoms akin to chronic fatigue syndrome pay to have injections of vitamin B12. However, without first establishing whether a deficiency of this vitamin occurs, it seems foolish to supplement with it given its proangiogenic properties. It also has implications for those with cancer and other medical conditions where angiogenesis is necessary for their development.

Many of the foods containing vitamin B12, such as liver, also contain excellent amounts of vitamin A which inhibit angiogenesis. This provides an inbuilt balance between a food containing nutrients which promote angiogenesis and those which inhibit it.

 However, it needs repeating that taking supplements of vitamin B12, without these being prescribed for a particular medical condition, may be unwise for those suffering from lipoedema or lipolymphoedema.

The lack of vitamin B12 in the vegetarian and vegan diet also raises questions as to whether those who follow these diets are actually less likely to develop psoriasis or - if they do - whether it progresses as quickly as those who are enthusiastic meat eaters and trying to determine what the picture is about.

Nevertheless, we do have some understanding of what happens in the progression and development of the condition and it is these areas that we can begin to tackle through a bespoke diet.

In The Journal of Functional Foods[2]: Vitamins and regulation of angiogenesis, Mohammed Al Saghiri et al have provided a helpful guide to foods that inhibit angiogenesis. This information is tabulated below.

Table showing anti- angiogenic vitamins and their mode of action.

Vitamin	inhibitory effect
Vitamin A	Suppresses VEGF
Vitamin B2 - riboflavin	Mechanism of inhibition not recorded
Vitamin B6	Inhibits microvascular outgrowth and suppresses the proliferation of endothelium cells

---

[2] Journal of Functional Foods: vitamins and regulation of angiogenesis. Mohammed Al Saghiri et al. Volume 38 Part A November 2017 pg. 180-196

Vitamin B9 – folic acid	Inhibits angiogenesis by decreasing endothelial cells and activating pathways that result in cell cycle arrest
Vitamin D	Anti-proliferative effects by inducing cell cycle arrest and apoptosis
Vitamin E - tocopherol	Inhibits proliferative tube formation of endothelial cells
Vitamin K	Inhibits VEGF

Table showing vitamins that inhibit angiogenesis and their food sources

Vitamin	Food Sources
Vitamin A- fat soluble vitamin – as such it should always be eaten with a little fat to aid its absorption	Found as a precursor in orange fruits and vegetables such as carrots. It is found in cod liver oil, liver, butter.
Vitamin B2* also	Found in milk,

known as riboflavin – water soluble	wholemeal bread and cereal, almonds, dark chicken meat and cooked beef
Vitamin B6 also known as niacin – water soluble	Pork, poultry, fish bread, wholegrain cereals, brown rice
Vitamin B9 – water soluble	Beans, citrus foods. Whole grain cereals, green leafy vegetables, beets, cauliflower, lettuce asparagus
Vitamin D – this is a fat soluble vitamin.	Main sources are sunlight, oily fish, eggs and irradiated mushrooms. However, it is unlikely that you can obtain all the vitamin D that you require from food sources
Vitamin E – fat soluble vitamin	Main sources are nuts, seeds and wheat germ
Vitamin K- fat soluble	There are two forms

vitamin	of vitamin K. One form is found in fermented food such as yogurt, cheese and soy sauce The second form is mainly found in dark green leafy vegetables

*Vitamin B is normally found in a complex and it is normally recommended that it is taken as such. However, as we are trying to utilise the inhibitory angiogenic properties of some of the B vitamins it is useful to know what their food sources are. It may be that single supplementation of vitamins B2, B6 and B9 may prove useful in preventing the manifestation of psoriasis.

On the subject of angiogenesis, I explained that the outcome of certain processes was T cell infiltration into psoriatic lesions. It may be helpful to explore T cells – cells of the immune system – in a little more detail to see how this comes about.

Naïve T helper cells differentiate into three different subsets known as:

- Th1
- Th2
- Th17

How they differentiate into one or another very much depends on the stimuli provided by cytokines.

Current ideas about psoriasis uphold the theory that there has initially to be a genetic predisposition to the condition.

A stimulus – as yet unknown – would interact with epidermal keratinocytes which would go onto produce substances known to be produced in the development of psoriasis.

These include:

- Tumour necrosis factor
- Interferon gamma

- Interferon alpha

Various other processes occur that result in the proliferation of skin cell known as epidermal hyper-proliferation. When this cell infiltration occurs with T cells (Th 17) then psoriatic lesions are manifested.

When we investigate the causes of new diseases, we can look at the environmental factors that exist at the time that appear to converge and result in a new condition. This is reasonably easy for fairly recent de novo conditions. It is far more difficult going back to the time of Hippocrates – when psoriasis was in existence – and trying to figure out what environmental factors may have contributed over such a lengthy period. Yes, there does appear to be a genetic predisposition but something has to turn those genes, for psoriasis on and off. I doubt very much that the main contender is lack of vitamin D. Psoriasis proliferates in Spain and Egypt just as much as it does in countries which have far less sunlight.

Maybe, just maybe, the answer partly lies in the balance of the angiogenic inhibitors and progressors in the diet that interact with specific genes. In effect a lack of angiogenic inhibitors would allow one of the processes found in the manifestation of psoriasis – that is angiogenesis - to flourish.

This would not be unreasonable given that proangiogenic and inhibitory angiogenic factors have existed over centuries and may be the one prevailing factor to account for psoriasis' long history.

Psoriasis sufferers are used to the relapsing and remitting nature of the condition. One lady I knew had psoriasis permanently from her early twenties which waxed and waned although she could never figure out why. When she was forty-five, the psoriasis disappeared and did not return for some years. It then returned to its former pattern. She noticed that, after eating, the psoriatic plaques would begin to itch, then burn to the extent that she either had to apply topical corticosteroid or scratch herself until she bled.

The psoriatic moratorium actually coincided with having a new partner who took over the cooking. As such, new dishes were introduced into her diet. When the relationship failed, she returned to her former diet. As she did so the psoriasis returned immediately. As this lady spent her life outdoors and spent many days in sunny climes, without any respite from this condition, I have to question whether a deficiency of vitamin D is contributing to the manifestation of this syndrome. There appears to be something that is dietary related and whose impact is more immediate.

Chronic inflammatory processes are at work in psoriasis which may be amenable to vitamin D supplementation where a deficiency occurs. Vitamin D does help to regulate the immune system controlling over activity.

Approximately 80% of the world population are deficient in this vitamin which is required for strong bones as well as regulating inflammation.

It is one of the most difficult of vitamins to take in sufficient quantities through the diet. Foods containing vitamin D are limited and what foods there are do not contain great amounts. As we get older we are less likely to absorb the nutrients from our diet. The absorbability of Vitamin D is no different. Therefore, increasing age is a risk factor for a deficiency of vitamin D.

Most of our vitamin D is taken in through the action of the sun's rays on the skin but even this process becomes less efficient as we age. Vitamin D is synthesised using the cholesterol found under the skin. Those on statins, therefore, may be vitamin D deficient, as their cholesterol levels have been artificially lowered.

Supplementation of 2000 IU's is recommended daily under a GP's supervision. The UK's recommended daily intake is 400 international units (IU's). However, this dose was set in the 1950's to prevent rickets from occurring which was rife at the time. This was the minimum amount that would prevent this condition from happening but not the amount that would provide overall optimum health.

This vitamin should be supplemented in the active form D3 rather than the inactive form, D2. The latter requires a number of steps to be converted to the active form. As age progresses, the conversion process is likely to be less effective.

Supplements are advised for

- The elderly
- Those who are housebound
- Those who work indoors
- Those with black skin
- Those with inflammatory bowel disease, or other conditions, where the ability to absorb nutrients is compromised.

Dietary sources of vitamin D are irradiated mushrooms, eggs and oily fish.

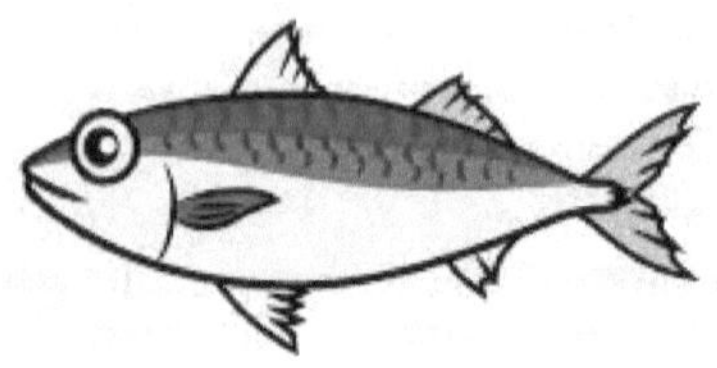

Oily fish such as mackerel, salmon and
fresh tuna contain good amounts of
vitamin D.

Cod liver oil is an excellent source of vitamin D if you can tolerate the taste.

Nevertheless, vitamin D is not the whole answer to the chronic inflammatory processes that occur with psoriasis. To look further into the subject of chronic inflammation it may be useful to look at the difference between acute and chronic inflammation before looking at some foods which are proinflammatory in nature, and further, are ubiquitous in the food chain. What you find may very well surprise you.

Acute and Chronic Inflammation

When tissue damage occurs due to injury or infection a whole set of processes occur involving the immune system. Various immune cells are sent to the site of injury or infection. Some cells - such as macrophages - that deal with infection or damaged cells, may phagocytose the debris. Others pour toxic substances on invading infections. Yet others may cause blood vessels to widen and become leaky in order to allow healing cells to travel to the site of injury.

When the infection has been dealt with and damaged tissue restored then the acute inflammatory processes will recede. Their job has now been done.

In some cases, this brake on inflammation does not occur. Inflammation becomes excessive and prolonged and is known as chronic inflammation.

Chronic inflammation is now known to be an underlying factor in most debilitating diseases.

Chronic inflammation produces lots of free radicals which then create more inflammation in the process. Chronic inflammation is like an out of control fire in your body. It is never quite quenched and continues to exert damage while it continues to smoulder.

Redness and heat which occur at the site of injury are due to increased blood flow to the site of inflammation. The swelling is caused by an accumulation of fluid. This presses on nerve endings causing pain.

Pain and itching is also due to the release of chemicals such as bradykinin and histamine that stimulate pain receptors.

Philip Schauer, MD, director of the Bariatric and Metabolic Institute at eh Cleveland Clinic stated, 'Chronic inflammation plays a direct role in diabetes, high blood pressure, sleep apnoea, asthma and other conditions.'

Antioxidants neutralise free radicals so that they can no longer cause damage and the subsequent inflammatory response. Antioxidants effectively put a brake on chronic inflammation and prevent the insidious and uncontrolled damage that is going on inside you.

The range of antioxidants is huge. The three main vitamins with antioxidant activity are

- Vitamin A and its precursor beta-carotene. Vitamin A is fat soluble and is found in liver, cheese, butter and oily fish. Its precursor is found in collards and orange coloured vegetables such as carrot and pumpkin.

- Vitamin C – vitamin C is found in fresh fruit and vegetables. It is water soluble and is easily destroyed by cooking. Most supermarkets have Vitamin C tablets which can be dropped into a glass of water and make a refreshing fizzy drink.

- Vitamin E – this is a fat soluble vitamin and is mainly found in nuts and wheat-germ. As high doses can cause bleeding then caution has to be applied if ibuprofen or some other NSAID is being taken alongside it as they can also create the tendency to bleed.

Lycopene is a bright red carotene found in tomatoes, papayas and watermelons. It also has antioxidant properties.

Dark chocolate, red wine, spices such as cinnamon and nutmeg and yellow mustard seed, can all be included in foods that have antioxidant properties.

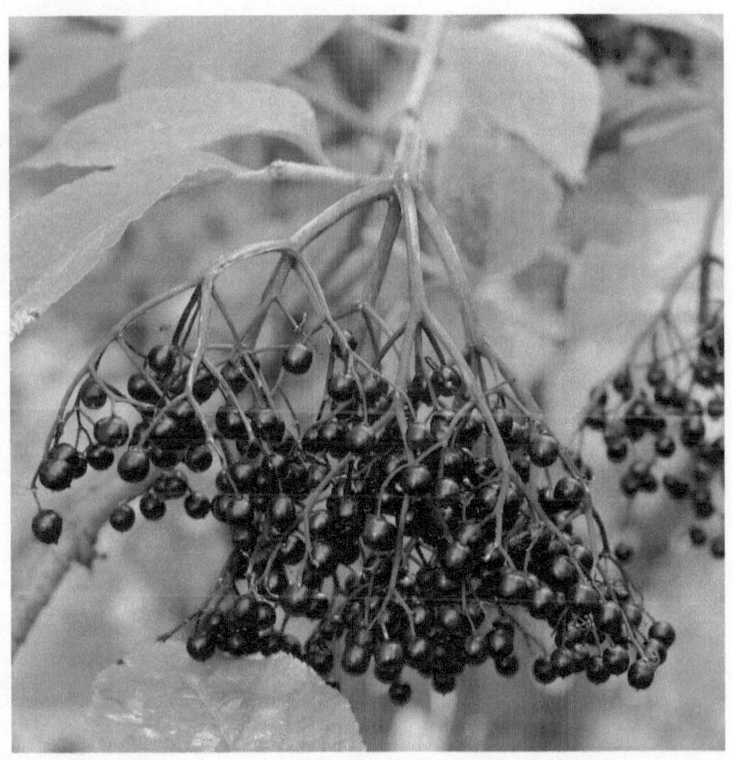

Nature produces an abundance of fruits and vegetables that are rich in antioxidants. This is why it is recommended that you include as many different colours and varieties of fruit and vegetables as possible in your diet.

Trace minerals as antioxidants.

The trace elements which are:
- Copper
- Selenium
- Manganese
- Zinc

act as co-factors of antioxidant enzymes to protect the body from oxygen free radicals. These oxygen free radicals are produced during oxidative stress.

Selenium, especially, tends to be deficient in many individuals. Many sources of selenium are dependent on the soil having adequate amounts of selenium within it which the plant will take into itself. Unfortunately, many soils suffer from selenium depletion. Nevertheless, two brazil nuts provide all the selenium that you require on a daily basis. Other good sources are mushrooms and brewer's yeast.

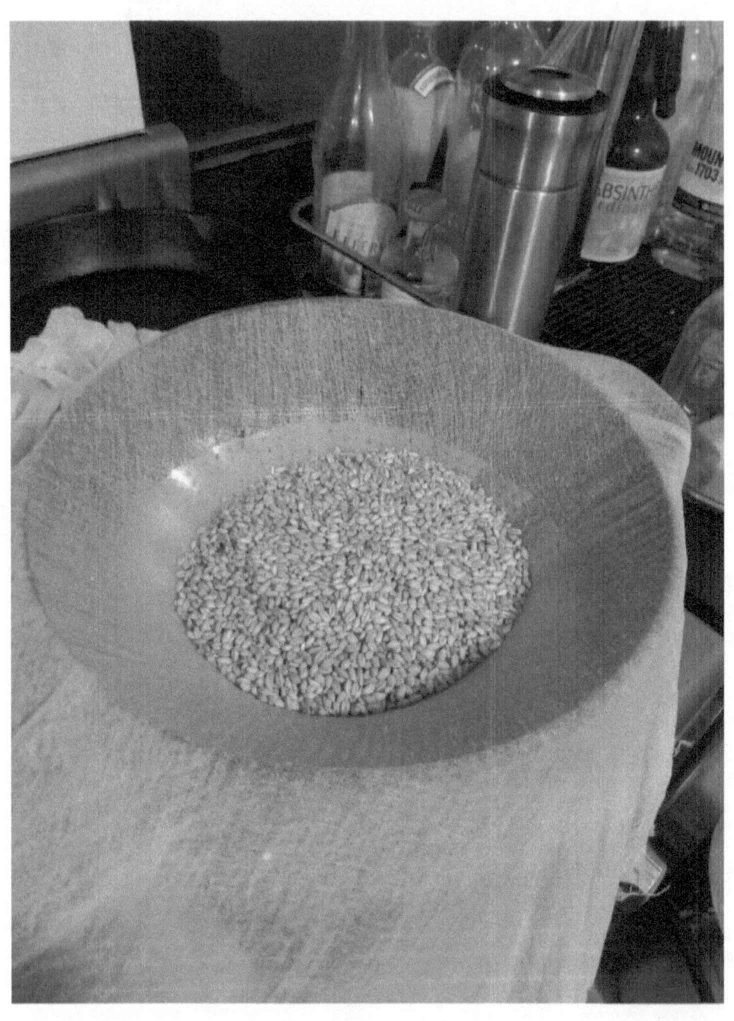

Brewer's yeast is a good source of selenium as well as the vitamin B complex

Selenium is often most severely deficient in those who are traumatised and receive parenteral micro-nutrition. Selenium assists the free radical scavenging activity of glutathione peroxidase as well as the immune system.

Good sources of copper are red meats especially offal. Supplementation of this trace element is not recommended. The copper found in meat is in a bound form – that is, it is attached to a protein source. Unbound copper such as that found in:

- Supplements
- Copper piping conveying water to households
- Copper bracelets

Is highly toxic to the brain. It slows down the removal of amyloid beta protein from the brain to the bloodstream. It is amyloid beta protein that is implicated in Alzheimer's disease.

The following foods are excellent sources of copper:[3]

	Amount	RDI
Beef liver, cooked	1 oz (28 g)	458%
Oysters, cooked	6	133%
Lobster, cooked	1 cup (145 g)	141%
Lamb liver, cooked	1 oz (28 g)	99%
Squid, cooked	3 oz (85 g)	90%
Dark chocolate	3.5 oz bar (100 g)	88%
Oats, raw	1 cup (156 g)	49%
Sesame seeds, roasted	1 oz (28 g)	35%
Cashew nuts, raw	1 oz (28 g)	31%

---

[3] https://www.healthline.com/nutrition/copper-deficiency-symptoms#section11

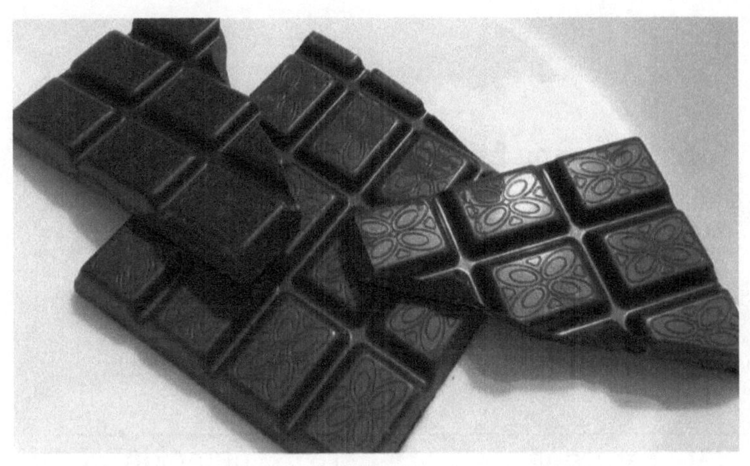

Dark chocolate contains useful amounts of copper

Good sources of manganese are lean meat, nuts, milk and seafood.

Table showing food sources of antioxidants

Antioxidant	Sources
Anthocyanins	Grapes, berries, aubergine
Sulphur compounds	Onions, leeks and garlic
Beta carotene	Carrots, pumpkin, mangoes, apricots, spinach and parsley
Catechins	Tea and red wine
Copper	Seafood, milk, nuts, meat, cocoa and dark chocolate
Cryptoxanthin	Mangoes, pumpkin, red pepper
Flavonoids	Tea, red wine, onion, apple, citrus fruit
Indoles	Cruciferous vegetables such as cabbage and cauliflower
Isoflavonoids	Lentils, peas, milk, tofu, soya products
Lignans	Bran, whole grains, vegetables, seeds

	such as linseed
Lutein	Leafy greens such as kale, chard and spinach
Lycopene	Tomatoes, pink grapefruit, watermelon
Manganese	Lean meat, nuts, milk, seafood
Polyphenols	Aromatic herbs such as thyme and oregano
Selenium	Brazil nuts (not more than two daily) seafood, whole grains organ meats
Vitamin C	Fresh fruit and vegetables
Vitamin E	Vegetable oils and whole grains. However, many vegetable oils create inflammation and are better avoided altogether. Olive oil, however, is a

	monounsaturated oil and is not proinflammatory in nature. This can be used freely. Keep it stored in the fridge in darkness.
Zinc	Nuts, milk, seafood and lean meat

The Role of Fasting in Reducing Chronic Inflammation

A recent article that appeared in the Medical Express has highlighted the importance of fasting in reducing inflammation and chronic inflammatory disease.

As we have already discovered lymphoedema is a chronic inflammatory disease which has the potential to respond to such measures. Even more exciting is the discovery that fasting does not affect the immune systems response to acute infections.

Calorie restriction has long been known to improve inflammatory and auto immune disease but how this comes about has only been discovered.

Apparently, intermittent fasting reduces the release of monocytes. These are pro-inflammatory cells which are found circulating in the blood. During fasting these cells go into a dormant state and become less inflammatory in the process.

Monocytes are highly inflammatory and can cause serious tissue damage. Dr Merad[4] explained that increasing amounts of monocytes can be seen in the blood circulation of populations, over the last few centuries, due to different eating patterns.

Moreover, in chronic psoriatic skin inflammation there is an increase in mono-adhesion and aggregation of monocytes. This is believed to be due to a monocyte dysfunction. When there is concomitant cardiovascular disease with psoriasis, there is a more severe outcome for patients. It is predictive of myocardial infarction and death.

---

[4] https://medicalxpress.com/news/2019-08-fasting-inflammation-chronic-inflammatory-diseases.html

Studies have shown that people who have a poor diet can ameliorate the effects by the periodic use of a low calorie, plant based diet. This causes the cells to act like the body is fasting.

Longo[5] and colleagues conducted clinical trials where participants were allowed to consume between 750and 1l00 calories daily over a five day period.   The diet contained specific proportions of proteins, fats and carbohydrates. The participants saw reduced risk factors for many life threatening diseases.

'Fasting is hard to stick to and it can be dangerous.   We know that the fasting-mimicking diet is safer and easier than water only fasting, but the big surprise from this study is that if you replace the fasting-mimicking diet, which includes pre-biotic ingredients, with water, we don't see the same benefits.

---

[5]

https://www.sciencedaily.com/releases/2019/03/190306171247.htm

In mice studies, these findings were replicated. In the study one group of mice adhered to a four-day fasting-mimicking diet by consuming approximately 50 percent of their normal caloric intake on the first day and 10 per cent of their normal caloric intake from the second through fourth days. Another group fasted with a water based diet only for 48 hours. The fasting-mimicking diet was found to mitigate or reverse some of the inflammatory processes while the water based fast did not. This indicated that certain nutrients in the fasting-mimicking diet contributed to the positive changes found in the plant based fast.

The conclusion formed was that 'fasting primes the body for improvement, but it is the re-feeding that provides the opportunity to rebuild cells and tissues.'

This is not the whole story about chronic inflammation though. Many studies have shown that the products of arachidonic acid known as 5-lipoxygenase are implicated in the pathophysiology of psoriasis.

The next chapter contains a little chemistry but explanations of some of the terms you may not have heard of, are given. It is a hugely important chapter to the understanding of the underlying pathological mechanisms of psoriasis and, as such, well worth reading. You may well be surprised at how ubiquitous arachidonic acid is, in our current diets, certainly more so since the beginning of the 20th century in respect of one newly introduced food. Nevertheless, arachidonic acid has been around since time immemorial in various forms.

It is to the subject of arachidonic acid - and 5-lipooxygenase - that we will now turn.

Arachidonic acid and 5-lipooxygenase

Arichidonic acid is a polyunsaturated omega-6 fatty acid. It is found in the membranes of the body's cells and is particularly abundant in the brain, muscles and liver. It is a key inflammatory intermediate and can act as a vasodilator. This means it can widen blood vessels. When blood vessels widen they may become leaky. This allows cells of the immune system through to deal with any areas infection or tissue damage.

Arachidonic acid promotes the growth and repair of muscle tissue via conversion to prostaglandins following exercise. It helps to promote muscle protein synthesis.

 In spite of the beneficial roles that arachidonic acid has in the body, it can cause inflammation when certain conditions occur.

However, this won't happen unless tiny particles, called electrons, try and disrupt the stability of other electrons found in the fat that forms part of the cell membranes.

Arachidonic acid, therefore, can be metabolised to both anti-inflammatory and proinflammatory eicanosoids.[6] It is quite likely that if you suffer from joint pain, bronchoconstriction, microvascular permeability and lymphoedema that arachidonic acid has been converted to a pro-inflammatory compound.

Eicanosoids are a class of compounds (like leukotrienes –see below - and prostaglandins)

---

[6] An eicanosoid is the end product of a process which help bring about inflammation.

which are synthesised from poly unsaturated fatty acids (PUFA's) - like arachidonic acid – and that are involved in cellular activity. They are lipid mediators of inflammation.

Leukotrienes

One of the end products of arachidonic acid is a white blood cell known as a leukotriene.

The biochemical definition of a leukotriene is:

Any of a group of biologically active compounds, originally isolated from leucocytes (white blood cells). They are metabolites of arachidonic acid, containing three conjugated bonds.

That's a bit of a mouthful so let's pull it apart and see what it really means.

A **leucocyte** is simply a white blood cell. They protect the body against infectious disease and foreign invaders.

A **metabolite** is the very end product of some chemical processes, that occur in a living organism, in order to maintain life.

Leukotrienes are the end product (metabolite) of **arachidonic acid.**

The negative effects of leukotrienes

The negative side effects of leukotrienes are generally known in association with asthma.

 Acute asthma attacks are often triggered by exercise or allergens. They are released by mast cells and are involved in bronchoconstriction. That is, they constrict the tubes that are found in the lungs that the passage of air travels along.

Leukotrienes also increase mucous secretion in both asthma and chronic obstructive pulmonary disease (COPD). In addition, they are implicated in the development of arthritis and atherosclerosis, as well as some cancers.

During the process of inflammation, leukotrienes also increase microvascular permeability.

The inflammatory processes of leukotrienes need to be targeted since it has been identified that it is this that contributes to the initiation, and progression, of psoriasis.

As we have learned that leukotrienes are the end product of arachidonic acid then we need to investigate the sources of this nutritional substance.

Sources of arachidonic acid

The sources of arachidonic acid are clearly important when it comes to investigating the causes of the chronic inflammatory processes that accompany psoriasis. A major source of arachidonic acid is derived from a group of poly unsaturated fatty acids (PUFA's) known as omega 6 fatty acids.

These are molecules that have some free 'arms.' They are unsaturated which also means they are unstable. Molecules do not like unpaired electrons and will take great pains to try and 'steal' electrons from other molecules causing damage – and consequently inflammation – in the process.

Our diets contain far greater amounts of omega 6's than ever before. They have replaced the stable – and largely unreactive - fats that we used to enjoy in the past.

The main stable fats that were used in developed countries were:

- Butter
- Dripping
- lard

Moreover, as we have replaced the stable fats with the potentially inflammatory omega 6 PUFA, we have also decreased the omega 3 PUFA which has known anti-inflammatory effects.

Omega 3 PUFA's are found oily fish such as mackerel, sardine and salmon. They are required in larger quantities than the omega 6 PUFA's but the ratio of omega 6 to omega 3 PUFA's is currently estimated at 6:1.

What are the main sources of omega 6 PUFA's?

 The main sources of omega 6 PUFA's are:

- Canola oil
- grapeseed oil
- corn oil
- soybean oil
- peanut oil

There are plenty of hidden sources of omega 6 PUFA's. Some unexpected sources are to be found in:

- Granola
- Crisps
- energy bars

- flax seeds
- commercially raised poultry, beef and eggs where corn is one of the main feeds.
- soup

The apparently healthy benefits of omega 6 PUFA's were heavily marketed in the 1970's in the UK. Omega 6 PUFA's do have healthy benefits when they are taken in moderation. However, the addition – and use - of these oils to most prepacked meals, biscuits and many other foods available in the supermarket and, in addition, the replacement of stable fats with these vegetable oils, has increased the potential for many inflammatory conditions –where there is a genetic propensity - to manifest themselves.

Table . Food sources of arachidonic acid (PFA 20:4), listed in descending order by percentages of their contribution to intake, based on data from the National Health and Nutrition Examination Survey 2005-2006

Rank	Food item	Contribution to intake (%)	Cumulative contribution (%)
1	Chicken and chicken mixed dishes	26.9	26.9
2	Eggs and egg mixed dishes	17.8	44.7
3	Beef and beef mixed dishes	7.3	52.0
4	Sausage, franks, bacon, and ribs	6.7	58.7
5	Other fish and fish mixed dishes	5.8	64.5
6	Burgers	4.6	69.1
7	Cold cuts	3.3	72.4
8	Pork and pork mixed dishes	3.1	75.5
9	Mexican mixed dishes	3.1	78.7
10	Pizza	2.8	81.5
11	Turkey and turkey mixed dishes	2.7	84.2
12	Pasta and pasta dishes	2.3	86.5
13	Grain-based desserts	2.0	88.5

Specific foods contributing at least 1% of eicosatetraenoic acid in descending order: shrimp and shrimp mixed dishes, soups, regular cheese

[7]

Oils which are rich in poly unsaturated fatty acids also generate aldehydes freely. Aldehydes

---

[7]

https://epi.grants.cancer.gov/diet/foodsources/fatty_acids/table4.html

are a significant health risk and help develop many conditions that involve oxidative stress. These include cancer, heart disease and dementia as well as psoriasis. In fact, the World Health Organisation found that aldehyde levels were found to be twenty times higher than the recommended level, in oils.

Aldehydes are also found in tobacco smoke, combustion engine exhaust fumes, in the manufacturing of resins and textiles, carpet manufacture and the making of leather goods to name but a few. It is interesting that there are higher rates of motor neuron disease in manufacturers of leather goods than any other occupation.

8

www.ncbi.nlm.nih.gov › pmc › articles › PMC5713437

These oils are also found in some extremely oxidant and biologically reactive compounds known as Advanced Glycation End products (AGE's).[8] These form through the oxidation of sugars, lipids and amino acids. These then form aldehydes which bind to proteins. It is this process that is thought to play a role in fuelling the inflammation found in psoriasis.

Are poly unsaturated fatty acids responsible for the chronic inflammation found in psoriasis? It is quite possible given that arachidonic acid is a PUFA and that its end product is the leukotriene B4 that has been found to be responsible for aspects of chronic inflammation found in many conditions.

Fortunately, for us, there are many 5-lipoxygenase inhibitors in the food chain. Most people will be eating some in their diet without realising the impact that these inhibitors can have on chronic inflammation. It is to the subject of 5-LO inhibitors that we will now turn

The role of 5-lipoxygenase inhibitors in the treatment of psoriasis

5-lipoxygenase (5-LO) is a key enzyme in the synthesis of leukotrienes. Its importance as a therapeutic target cannot be underestimated.

5-LO brings about the first two steps of the transformation of arachidonic acid to leukotrienes.

 However, the only clinically approved inhibitor of 5-lipoxygenase – zileuton – has unacceptable side effects. These include:

- nausea
- upset stomach
- diarrhoea
- trouble sleeping
- headache
- myalgia
- sinus pain and symptoms often associated with colds

The good news is that there are some naturally occurring 5-lipoxygenase inhibitors. These include:

- Caffeic acid phenpropyl ester (found in bee propolis)
- Diphenlethyl ester*
- Phenylpropyl*
- Hypericum perforatum
- Gamma tocotrienol
- Delta tocopherol
- Gamma tocopherol
- Curcumin
- Erucic acid
- Monoenoic fatty acids
- Pumpkin seeds

We shall look at these – and others - in more detail later.

The starred substances above were found[9] to be significantly greater in inhibitory action than the reference molecules – which also showed 5-

---

lipoxygenase inhibitory action. These included caffeic acid phenyl ester (CAPE) and zileuton.

 Honey bee propolis is a good source of CAPE. Honey bee propolis exerts a number of beneficial effects. These include:

- Anti-inflammatory action
- Antiviral
- Anticancer
- Antibacterial

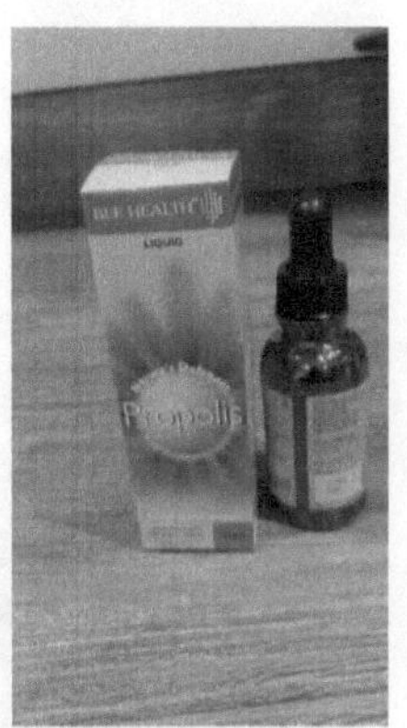

Monoenoic fatty acids

A number of long chain monoenoic fatty acids were found to have an effect on 5-LO activity. The results [10]show that oleic acid found in olive oil has by far the greatest inhibitory effect on 5-LO. Oleic acid is a monounsaturated fatty acid that is found in goodly amounts in olive oil and macadamia nuts.

Effect of Fatty Acid Inhibition Relative to Position of the Point of Unsaturation

Fatty acid	2.5	5.0	10	20	Chain length	Terminal	Carboxyl
	Inhibition (%) ----------(μmoles)----------					Number of carbons from double bond to:	
Oleic	48	66	77	89	18	9	9
Ricinoleic	17	35	67	90	18	9	9
Petroselinic	25	44	67	84	18	12	6
Vaccenic (*cis*)	40	70	83	92	18	7	11
5-*cis*-Eicosenoic	0	1	4	37	20	15	5
11-*cis*-Eicosenoic	25	40	62	81	20	9	11
Erucic	21	40	66	88	22	9	13
Nervonic	68	74	83	91	24	9	15

It is no hardship using olive oil in salad dressings, pouring a tablespoon over meals or dipping a sandwich in a small amount before eating.

---

[10] https://link.springer.com/article/10.1007%2FBF02534605

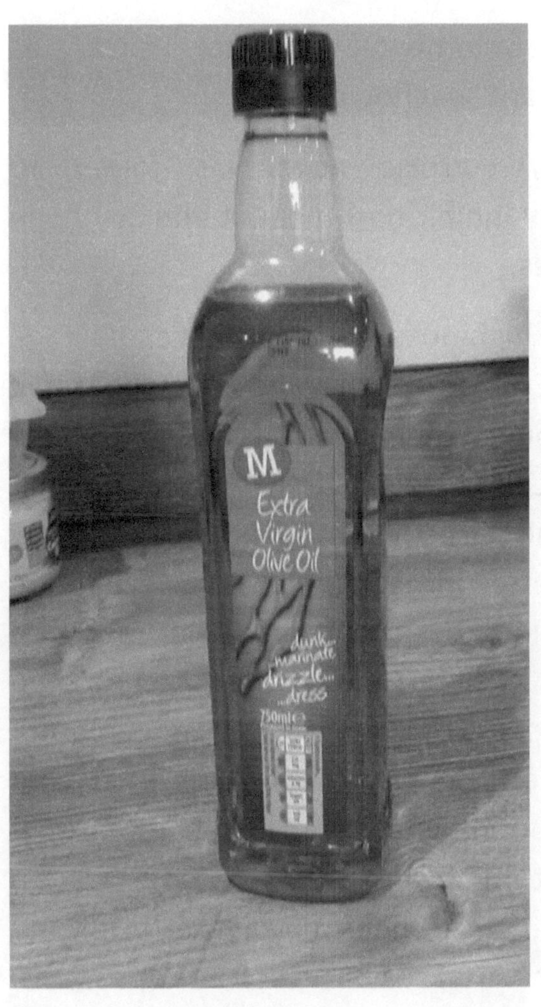

Erucic acid – a monoeic fatty acid - is found in rapeseed oil, mainly. However, it is also found in many ornamental flowers such as nasturtiums and wallflowers.

In a study[11] erucic acid was found to competitively inhibit both peanut and soy bean lipoxygenases.

However, at high doses, erucic acid can damage the heart. Erucic acid may be eaten in small amounts though. Indeed, as it is added to many takeaway, ready meals and snacks, it is difficult to avoid and already forms a part of many people's diets, unwittingly or not. What we need to avoid is the excessive use of rapeseed oil because of this. I would even go one step further and state that due to the inflammatory effects of the PUFA's they should be used with extreme caution, if at all. The liberal use of them, in just about any prepared food, has the potential for cancer, heart disease, arthritis and many other diseases as well as psoriasis.

11

https://onlinelibrary.wiley.com/doi/pdf/10.1007/BF02534605

by AJ St. Angelo - 1984

Moderation is the key. However, when a new product is marketed as being healthy the tendency is that manufacturers of products add it – quite unnaturally - to just about everything.

Many keen gardeners will know the ease with which nasturtiums can grow. In fact, the poorer the soil, the better. All parts of the nasturtium are edible including leaves, flowers and seeds. They look good tossed in salads and impart a peppery fresh flavour to the salad bowl. These are potentially a good source of erucic acid if you

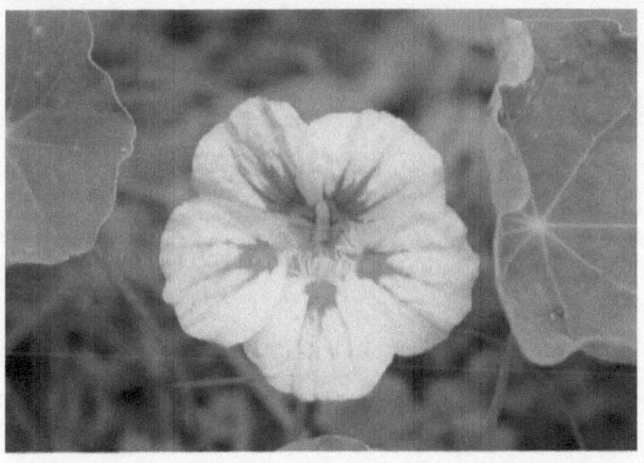

Nasturtiums come in a wide range of cheerful colours.

do not eat a diet that is already full of it and you wish to add a little as a 5-LO inhibitor.

Gamma tocotrienol, delta tocopherol and gamma tocopherol are different forms of vitamin E. Good sources of vitamin E are:

- Nuts and nut oils
- Seeds
- Wheat germ

Sources of vitamin E have a tendency to oxidise rapidly. Therefore, they are better stored in a cool dark place and eaten fairly soon after purchase.

The role of desaturase enzymes in chronic inflammation

Desaturase enzymes are rife in the development and progression of chronic inflammation so it may be prudent to ascertain what they are and, how they contribute to chronic inflammation.

These enzymes have a dual function. They are able to convert fatty acids to either pro inflammatory or anti-inflammatory products. As Inflammation helps us repair and heal - at times of injury or illness – then clearly we need desaturase enzymes to convert fatty acids into pro inflammatory substances are required for this purpose. However, when injury or illness is absent, then the conversion of fatty acids to anti-inflammatory products is the desired outcome.

Desaturase enzymes, however, require a number of essential nutrients in order to respond appropriately to the body's status. These are included for convenience in the box below.

What are desaturase enzymes?

Desaturase enzymes help produce and convert fatty acids to their preferred end product- that is, either anti-inflammatory or proinflammatory mediators. These enzymes cannot carry this task out in isolation. For example,

Delta 5-desaturase requires, niacin, zinc and vitamin C

Delta 6-saturase requires enough magnesium, B6 and zinc to function properly.

Zinc deficiency is rare in the developed world but may happen in someone with a poor diet.

Magnesium deficiency is quite common – more so if diuretics or laxatives are taken. Indeed, a study argued that subclinical magnesium deficiency is a public health crisis and may affect 80 of the population.

Those people who do not eat a diet with nuts or wholegrains are likely to be vitamin B6 deficient. Vitamin B6 is a water soluble vitamin and easily leaches into cooking water. In addition, it is easily destroyed by heat.

Any one of the above deficiencies can help to progress psoriasis

Zinc, magnesium and vitamin B6 (the latter is better taken in a complex of B vitamins) may all be supplemented. They can generally be obtained at local supermarkets and therefore do not generally cost much. If not, then they may be obtained at health stores or online.

Good sources of zinc include:

- seeds
- meat
- shellfish
- beans, chickpeas, lentils and other legumes

- eggs
- whole grains
- nuts
- dairy

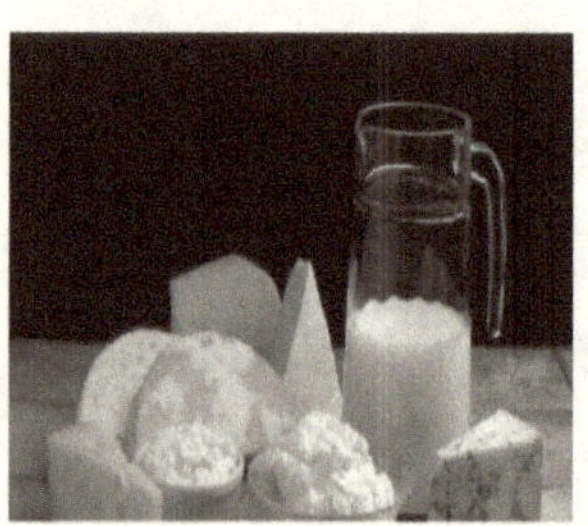

**Dairy foods
are a good
source of zinc**

The recommended dietary allowances of these nutrients are:

Zinc: 11mg for men, 8mg for women

Magnesium: 500mg

Vitamin B6: 1.5mg for women, 2mg for men

*[12]Vitamin C: 30mg

---

[12] I would query whether the RDA of 30mg for vitamin C is enough. I would recommend at least 100mg daily – certainly more for smokers and those living near environmentally polluted places.

Using Dimethyl sulfoxide (DMSO) as a therapy for chronic inflammation in resistant psoriasis

DMSO is a prescription medicine and dietary supplement, with powerful anti-inflammatory properties that can be used topically or taken by mouth. In some cases, it is given intravenously.

It has efficacy in many conditions –including psoriasis – and can decrease pain and speed the healing of tissue injury.

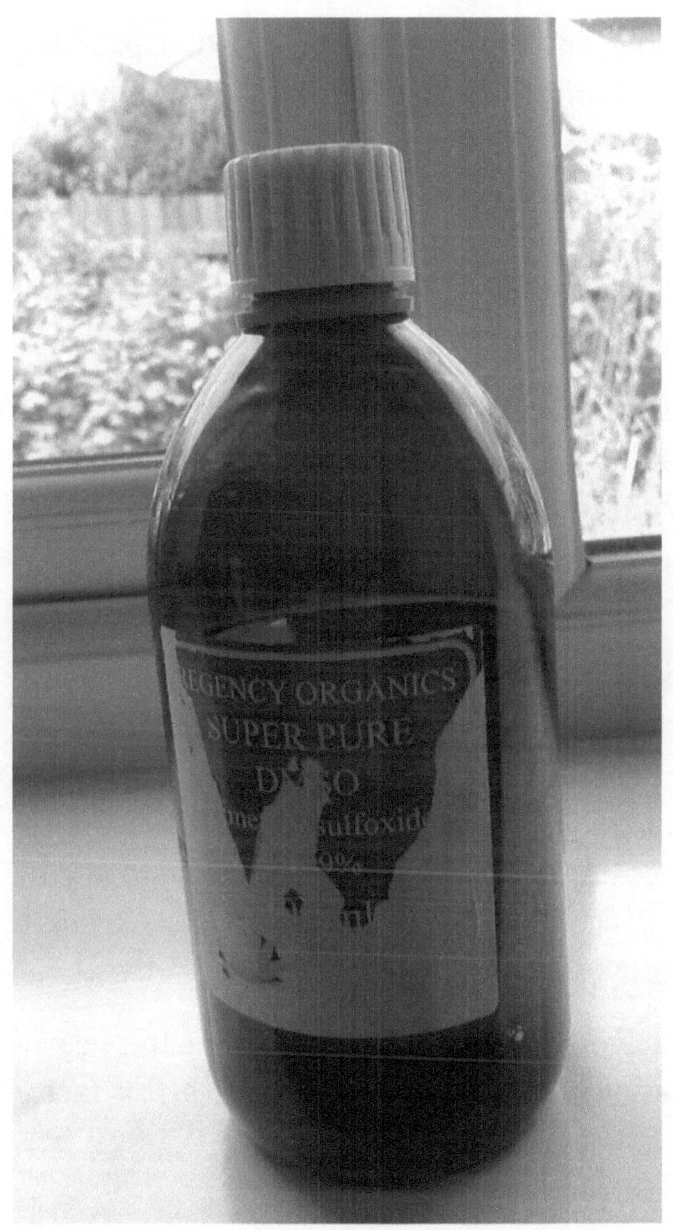
REGENCY ORGANICS
SUPER PURE
DMSO
Dimethyl sulfoxide
100%

A paper entitled **Therapy of resistant psoriasis with topical corticosteroids and dimethyl sulfoxide**[13] by Kaidbey KH found that the sequential application of full-strength dimethyl sulfoxide and potent topical corticosteroid preparations was very effective in resistant plaque-type psoriasis.

It was found that complete clearing could be obtained in 3-4 weeks. Lower strength DMSO was not found to be effective.

The use of DMSO can produce some stinging and burning on skin whether on psoriatic plaques or healthy skin. The use of topical corticosteroids limited these symptoms to transient burning or stinging, according to the research. Therefore, when resistance to topical corticosteroids occurs, this may be overcome by the concomitant use of topical full strength dimethyl sulfoxide.

Some research has highlighted that the use of dimethyl sulfoxide appears to be a risk factor

---

[13] https://www.ncbi.nlm.nih.gov/pubmed/955230

for cataracts in dogs. However, DMSO is used to treat cataracts and glaucoma in humans.

It is not clear when the canine research can be extrapolated to humans but while not impossible it is unlikely.

Eicosapentaenoic acid as a steroid substitute

Earlier in this book I stated that we had an imbalance of omega 6 and omega 3 fatty acids in the diet. Omega 6 PUFA's are proinflammatory and omega 3 PUFA's are anti-inflammatory in nature.

One of the omega 3 PUFA's which is relevant to the subject of psoriasis is eicosapentaenoic acid (EPA).

EPA inhibits the enzyme that helps synthesise arachidonic acid. The more EPA that you have in your diet the less arachidonic acid you will synthesise. In effect EPA reduces the amount of arachidonic acid and consequently the pro-inflammatory, prostaglandins, thromboxanes, eicosanoids and leukotrienes.

 the less arachidonic acid you will synthesise. In effect EPA reduces the amount of arachidonic acid and subsequently the pro-inflammatory prostaglandins, thromboxanes, eicosanoids and leukotrienes.

DHA, another omega three fatty acid and closely associated with EPA does not have this effect. It is not an inhibitor of the D5D enzyme. It has a greater spatial size and cannot compete with arachidonic acid for the enzyme phospholipase A2 that helps release arachidonic acid from the cell membrane phospholipids where it is stored. Only EPA can do this.

 Interestingly, steroid therapy generally inhibits this D5D enzyme to reduce inflammation. However, EPA can do this but without the numerous side effects of steroids.

The main source of EPA is oily fish such as salmon, pilchards, mackerel and sardines. Oily fish needs to be eaten daily when psoriasis is present.   Failing this, supplementation is necessary as a preventative step   in inhibiting the D5D enzyme that is necessary for the synthesis of arachidonic acid.

How Iron status affects the development of psoriasis

A number of fairly recent pieces of research have raised the issue that deranged iron status, especially in those with low body mass, contributes to the development and severity of psoriasis.

Iron deficiency is well known to aggravate inflammatory mediated chronic disorders, a description which fits psoriasis well. Conversely, such chronic inflammatory mediated disorders tend to result in iron deficiency

Iron deficiency has an adverse effect on the function of immune system cells and thus can contribute to disease progression.

In one study, a number of biomarkers of iron status were measured in 39 patients with psoriasis in 17 men ranging from 37-57 years and 44 healthy subjects of which 30 were men ranging from 47-59 years.

The results showed that compared to healthy controls, the patients with psoriasis had a similar blood status but they did show a deranged iron status. Nevertheless, the status of the biomarkers did not really reflect the severity of the disease. However, what was ultimately revealed was that there was a significant correlation of the severity of the disease with low body mass index.

The conclusion of the study was that there was a significant correlation between psoriasis and deranged iron status (that is, depleted iron stores) which is aggravated in those with a lower body mass index.

While most people believe that psoriasis only affects the skin it is a much more complex condition with many 'under the surface' abnormalities going on which include autoimmune responses and the activation of pro-inflammatory immune system cells which impact all body organs and tissues.

It appears that iron status is vital in instructing the immune cells – which belong to the innate immune system - to function correctly. Aberrations in the innate immune system lend to the manifestation of chronic inflammatory conditions such as CKD and rheumatoid arthritis.

Sometimes, it is an overexpression of an iron biomarker, hepcidin, which causes the problem. Excess hepcidin occurs when proinflammatory cytokines are manifest because the iron then becomes trapped inside cells and so is unavailable for use by the body.

It follows, then, that there are two mechanisms by which iron derangement may occur and these are:

Iron deficiency anaemia with an emphasis on low body mass or

An over expression of hepcidin occurring as a results of pro-inflammatory markers.

In the latter case there are many natural immunosuppressant's which are originated from plant sources. Many of these are already well known and include: resveratrol, piperine, curcumin and luteolin. Not only do they inhibit the production of these pro-inflammatory cytokines but they also inhibit the release. Inhibition is generally achieved by altering the signalling pathways which enable the production and release of these chemicals

Vitamin D   has a major impact on the modulation of the innate immune system as we have already seen. Vitamin D deficiency is rife and needs to be corrected. Additionally, vitamin C has excellent value in suppressing rogue pro-inflammatory action.

Of course, not all inflammation is bad. We need pro-inflammatory action when the body needs to fight infection or repair itself but all too often, when the repair is completed or the infection has been dealt with, the body does not appear to recognise this and continues with its pro-inflammatory action. When it is not needed, it is damaging.

There are many causes of the acute phase inflammation which leads to the increase in hepcidin. These include allergens, irritants, toxic compounds. The latter is often found as adjuvants added to flu jabs and similar but is not confined to this by any means.

Foreign bodies that damage the macrophages because they are too large to be phagocytosed by them will also induce an inflammatory response. There are many such foreign bodies in our environment such as asbestos and silica. While many will be familiar with the dangers of asbestosis, awareness of the problems surrounding silica are less well known.

While silica in the right place has benefits for skin and hair, in the wrong place it can be fatal.

Silica dust abounds in workplaces involved with construction elements such as sand, clay, ceramics and bricks. The dust is deadly and symptoms of silicosis include a persistent cough and shortness of breath. The lung inflammation is deep caused by fine dust particles which are also known as reparable crystalline silica.

It can be understood that conditions which do not appear to be connected may impact the manifestation of another and the latter is unlikely to clear up until the former is addressed.

We are living in a toxic environment. There is no doubt about that and there may be many such toxic events that need to be investigated and addressing before psoriasis can be eliminated.

However, we need to turn to simple iron deficiency anaemia which is rife in society given the number of plant based diets which are associated with iron deficiency anaemia. Iron from plants is lacking –compared to animal sources – and it is also poorly absorbed requiring vitamin C to be present at the same time. No such requirement is needed for the more bioavailable form of iron found in cuts of meat. Liver, of course, is an excellent source of iron but has fallen out of favour since the immediate post war years.

Sadly, red meat has been demonised thus potentially contributing to the increase in pro-inflammatory conditions such as chronic kidney disease through iron deficiency.

While anaemia and its impact was well known and identified in the 1950's when I grew up as a child, it is thought to be almost eliminated due to our 'good diets.'   I hear a lot of people talking about their 'good diets' while nibbling on a lettuce leaf and apologising if their diet goes much beyond that. This self-flagellation when it comes to food needs to stop.   We do not grow healthy on limiting our diets to pasta and salads with a sugar free yogurt for dessert.

Perhaps we need to go back to first principles and learn about iron.

Iron exists as ferrous iron and ferric iron. It is an essential trace mineral where approximately is present as haemoglobin. This is the red pigment of the blood which carries oxygen around the body. The rest is stored in the liver, bone-marrow, muscles, as myoglobin, and spleen.

Losses of about 1mg occur daily and these are brought about by menstruation, breastfeeding and some is lost by the normal breakdown of blood. It can be seen from this that iron deficiency anaemia is more likely to occur in women and it is well researched that psoriasis is rifer in women than men.

Iron absorption is always higher in children and this phenomenon reduces in later years. Thus, a reduction in the haem form (animal protein) which is more bioavailable is not always wise as a person ages.

Meat sources of iron tend to be discarded due to the fact that older people find it more difficult to chew. Buying minced varieties or long slow cooking will prevent meat from being rejected.

Deficiency symptoms are many and include:

Tiredness

Lack of stamina

Pallor

Breathlessness

Giddiness

Headaches

Insomnia

Palpitations

anxiety

hair loss and thinning

brain fog

While it is fairly easy to test for iron deficiency, this isn't always undertaken with the enthusiasm it could be. Many people are finding it quite difficult to access medical care. If we go back to the older medicine, the lower eyelid was simply retracted gently and if the inner eyelid was not a bright rich red but leaned towards peach or lemon, then the individual was deemed to be anaemic. Of course, this did not supply the cause but if we start off with the most likely cause then it is poor diet and/or absorption and needs to be corrected.

On meeting up with two friends, aged 88 and 90 years who had been complaining of fatigue, I asked them to retract their lower eyelid to find that both had completely white lower inner eyelids with a small reddish blood vessel making an appearance. I informed them immediately that I was not surprised they were fatigued and suggested that they get some non-constipating iron.

I, prior to that, having been busy for prolonged periods and abandoning my meat rich diet found that a couple of irritating psoriatic patches had returned. On examining my own inner eyelid, I felt that I needed to follow my own advice and took a course of the same iron that I had suggested whereupon the psoriasis disappeared. I shall now use that symptom as a potential timely warning that I need to look at my iron levels.

Fortunately, iron has a number of best food sources which include these amounts per 100mg

Cockles 33.0

Dried brewer's yeast 20.0

Winkles 15.1

Wheat bran 12.8

Cooked liver 12.5

Cooked kidney 11.5

Cocoa powder 10.5

Soya flour 8.0

Parsley 8.0

Dried fruits 5.8

Sardines 4.1

Cereals 4.0

Corned beef 2.8

Wholemeal bread 2.5

Haricot beans 2.5

Beef 1.9

But bear in mind that the iron in beef is far more bioavailable than will be found in plant based foods.

The recommended daily intake is 10-12mg for children and 15-18mg for adults. A quick top up over 3 days or so will probably reveal the potential for iron deficiency anaemia.

A word of caution here- while shell fish is an excellent source of iron, it is also an excellent source of copper and copper in some susceptible people may increase the severity of psoriasis. However, this would be through a different mechanism and is unlikely to occur unless you had been dealt a double whammy: - that of a propensity to psoriasis through a vulnerability to iron deficiency and a genetic propensity to increased copper load. Some people appear to store copper better and others just have preference for foods which just happen to contain copper.

Happily, iron is able to reduce the absorption of copper as it can zinc. Indeed, these three can inhibit each other but which comes out top dog and gets to inhibit the others is a matter of genetics.

With any distressing condition like psoriasis, it does pay to undertake a little research to find out the potential culprits, one by one, and eliminate them when necessary.

Another little known side effect of poor iron status is generalised itching. Many people think they have suddenly developed an allergy but this cannot be further from the truth.   Again, using the lower inner eyelid test can be very revealing and indicate which treatment is necessary.

Iron excess is also harmful and needs to be avoided. Judicious use of iron is the key. If a GP is not available to take a blood test for anaemia, then there are many cheap and useful tests to be found in the chemist or online. Nevertheless, the eyelid test still carries revealing convenience and should not be thought of as carrying less importance.

Final Thoughts

There is no doubt that psoriasis is a debilitating and oft disfiguring condition that has a long history. While there may be a genetic propensity to this condition, genes do not have the final say in whether the condition is manifested or not. The deciding factor is undoubtedly the presence of various environmental factors, including diet, that can progress or inhibit processes like chronic inflammation or angiogenesis that are characteristic of this condition.

Dietary factors do not appear to be given huge amounts of consideration in the development and progression of psoriasis. I can understand why. It is after all a huge and complex subject to cover – if it can indeed ever be covered in its entirely. Nevertheless, dietary substances provide an almost endless array of treatments without the side effects that conventional medicines often carry, provided that they are not taken to excess through the unwise use of numerous food items that contain them as additives.

It can be seen that the eggs from corn fed chickens will be pro-inflammatory in nature while those chickens allowed to roam free will produce eggs that have anti-inflammatory properties. Corn oil is hugely inflammatory in nature but corn also contains a substance known as lutein which is eye protective. This demonstrates how a well-balanced diet that includes a diverse range of foods from both plant and animal sources is necessary for health.

Families are using more ready meals than ever before either through lack of time or lack of skills.

Cookery skills have largely been taken off the school curriculum. In households, where two parents are working, there is often little input into food preparation. The role of vitamins and minerals and the essential part that they play in health is conspicuous by their absence in education. Grandparents often have a major role to play in the education of their grandchildren but the closely knit family ties have largely been eroded through geographical distance and family breakdown.

Psoriasis does appear to have a genetic component to it. Passing on vital knowledge about the underlying processes of psoriasis and, just as importantly, what works to alleviate it, is vital.

Many skin conditions, including psoriasis, are not always given the importance, or understanding, that they deserve in medicine. It is therefore necessary for sufferers of psoriasis to learn self-management of this condition that includes the importance of dietary strategies that will help alleviate this condition.

Thank you for purchasing this book. Every time a book is purchased, a donation is made to one of the charities I am currently supporting.
These can be found on my author's website.
See below.

Other Health Related Books by the Author

- **The Reluctant Bowel**
- **A Weighty Issue**
- **Sleep, Perchance to Dream**
- **The Journey: EDS and chronic pain**
- **The MND diet: using nutrition to slow down the progress of neurodegeneration**
- **A Necessary Sorrow**
- **Treat infection Naturally**
- **Successful Aging**
- **Taking another Road: Pain: its causes and what can be done about it**
- **Osteoarthritis and Pain**
- **A Treatment Strategy for Migraine**

These can be found here on the author's page

https://www.amazon.co.uk/-/e/B07BPQZ5CD

You may also be interested in the semi-autobiographical trilogy of the authors life found in these three books

- The Prejudged
- Where the Blackbird Never Sings
- A Summer's Symphony

And the author's children's books

- Fanny and Victorian Jack
- Fanny and the Gamekeeper's Cottage

May I also make a plea that if you have enjoyed this book and benefitted from it that you would leave a review. Only one in two hundred readers, approximately, will leave a review for any book but reviews are important to authors. Thank you.

9 798616 673169